Not Dead Yet

A practical guide for the dying and those
who are supporting them.

Amanda Collins

First published by Busybird Publishing 2019
Large Print Edition 2020
Copyright © 2019 Amanda Collins

PRINT: 978-1-922465-02-3

Cover image: Kev Howlett

Cover design: Busybird Publishing

Layout and typesetting: Busybird Publishing

busybird
publishing

Busybird Publishing
2/118 Para Road
Montmorency, Victoria
Australia 3094
www.busybird.com.au

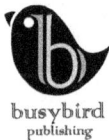

For Dave, who knows.

In memory of Robin Collins, my darling Dad,
who was sure there was a better way.

You were right, Dad.

Contents

Well hello.

Thank you for picking up this book – I hope it will give you a lot of support. Whether you just know you are going to die some day, or whether you have been 'moved up the queue' a bit, you will find some practical suggestions to help you cope with what can be a difficult time for you and your family.

A death can be a very tough time for carers, but it can also be an opportunity for some of the most special moments of kindness, respect and support.

A word on family – I speak a lot about family in this book and I want you to know that you don't need to share any genetic material with your loved ones to make them family. Often the best family is the one you choose to surround yourself with.

A word on death itself – nobody knows for certain what happens after you die. The part you have a say in is **right now** – your life. I'd like to encourage you to live that life to the fullest. How that might look will be different for everyone. But please, as you're considering your death, don't forget to LIVE.

In this book you will find:

- *Support for carers and those who are actively dying*

- *Suggestions for how to have the difficult conversations*
  - *With those you love*
  - *With medical staff*
  - *With children*

- *Help making the tough decisions*
  - *On living*
  - *On dying*
  - *On everything in between*

Everyone is different

It really is as simple, and as complicated, as that. Everyone has their own ideas about death, from suspicions to firmly held convictions, and everyone will approach it in their own way.

Some people will go to great lengths to NOT approach death. For these folk, even discussing death is too hard. If this is you, thank you for even reading this far. If you can, please find someone to talk it over with. There are many ways to make dying more comfortable and less terrifying, and these are worth finding out about.

Death cafés are currently in vogue, and provide an opportunity for people to discuss death and dying without any agendas or financial motivations. You can find more about local death cafés online.

Death doulas are becoming more commonly available, and they, along with many counsellors, are well versed in discussing death and dying options. At the end of this book I have listed several excellent online resources, which can also be a good place to start.

Having an advance care directive, a legal will and other legacy documents are so important, not only for your peace of mind, but also to help the people who will want to help you – whether that's your family, friends or health professionals.

Bill was a healthy 47-year old. With his own parents in good health, he had never seen the need to discuss dying or advance care options with his family. Most of all, he didn't want to make them feel uncomfortable or awkward, so he left the topic well alone. When a debilitating illness left him comatose and unable to communicate, he wasn't able to let them know what he would have preferred in terms of treatment options. They didn't know whether he would want months of rehab and invasive medical treatments, or whether he would have preferred to die gently in hospital over several days.

How do I know what I want when it comes to death?

Some questions for you to consider talking about with those you love:

What are your beliefs around health care? Quality of life? Prolonging life? Ending life?

Whose opinions do you value? Who gets a say in how your last days are conducted? If you are unable to speak up, who do you want to speak on your behalf?

Who do you know of who had a 'good death'? What did that look like?

What are your family's beliefs around these issues and do they match with yours? Now is the perfect time to find out. Put the kettle on, serve the ice cream or crack open a beer and talk.

Finding a good friend, a counsellor or a death doula who can talk these questions through with you can be immensely helpful. Even writing the answers in a journal will help you tease out what really matters to you.

What does a death doula do?

Much as a midwife can support a woman giving birth, a death doula assists people in all aspects of their death and dying. They come from many different backgrounds, and all offer great support to those who are dying and their families. Just as choosing a midwife is an individual preference, choosing a death doula will depend upon your family and their preferences.

'When I got "the diagnosis", my sister recommended a local death doula. She has been a great sounding board for the whole family, and has been able to sit with us on some of the tougher days. When I was going through a bad patch recently, we hired her to be present with me during the evening hours so my partner could get the kids to bed and make it

to the gym which was such a sanity saver. She has so many contacts and understands how this whole death thing works. And she's not judgemental. She just fit right in with our family when we needed her. I'm doing all right at the moment, but I know when it gets bad again, we can call on her to give the rest of my family a break. She will be there right through to the time I go to the undertaker.'
– Sandra, 47

Who gets a say?

Dear dying person,

This is your call. Your. Call. You might like to ask for advice from trusted friends, life partners, family members, health professionals or spiritual advisors, but in the end – with some good planning and a little luck – you can get to choose how you are cared for as you die.

We all like to think that we are in control of our lives, but death really does remove that illusion. Having discussed the possibilities around your death – from 'how will it most likely happen?' to 'what and who I want around me when I die' – will help each and every one of us feel a little more in control.

If you're caring for someone who is dying, be guided by them. Not just what you think they might want, but ASK them what they want. While you can. Have that talk, whether it's over a nice glass of wine, on a car ride somewhere or while looking at the stars.

The only person who really needs to be consulted is the person doing the dying; if they have managed to get all of their ducks in a row and assemble a team around them to gently support them.

People turn up at different stages when a person is dying. If preferences have been discussed, and plans are in place, when a new carer arrives, the advocates for the dying person will be able to gently steer well-meaning new arrivals into activities that contribute to everyone's well-being.

The imminent death of a loved one can drastically change family dynamics. You may have been 'picking up the slack' for a long time, or you may have not been involved at all. Either way, be aware that the situation has now changed, and others may want to be more involved than previously, or may expect your involvement.

If you have been the primary caregiver, please take good care of yourself – more on this below. Please remember, you can't do it all, and it's healing and comforting to let others be involved.

What to say
(when no-one is saying it)

Talking about dying when it's happening to you

You will find that some medical practitioners are very practiced at talking about death and dying, and some really struggle.

It's not your job to make the latter feel better, so, if you can, find someone else to talk to, who will answer your questions honestly.

It's OK to ask:

- *Am I dying?*
- *How long do you think I have until I die?*
- *How much worse is it going to get?*
- *What do you expect will happen over the next few months?*

- *How long will I have any quality of life for?*
- *What changes will happen in my body?*
- *What do other people do in this situation?*
- *What support is available, both privately and publicly funded?*

A note on asking these questions – some people choose not to ask, because they have found that getting specific answers can limit their outlook, and their capacity to live full lives, for however long that might be. The important thing is that you have the right to ask the questions you want answers to.

Talking about dying when it's happening to someone you love

If someone you know has had 'the diagnosis', our culture has a very limited palette of appropriate comments. The number of people who tell me they received 'Get Well Soon' cards when they tell friends and family that their condition is terminal is astonishingly high.

<u>*Some things NOT to say (PLEASE):*</u>

- *I know someone who had your condition and they went to Thailand/California/Iceland for a miracle cure, you should try it.*

- *I read about your condition on Facebook/Google, and here's my opinion.*

- *Chin up.*

- *It could be worse.*

<u>*Some things you COULD say instead:*</u>

- *Do you want to talk about it? (And it's OK if they don't want to)*

- *Where are you at today?*

- *What kind of support are you getting?*

- *What kind of support do you need? (And then follow through!)*

One of the worst things about being so sick is the way it rules your life. No-one wants to spend their waking hours dissecting their illness ... so be prepared to talk about normal life and what's going on in the world. How the person is feeling on a given day will dictate how engaged they want to be.

The world will still have its share of news and current affairs, sports and celebrity gossip. Talk about the things that interest the two of you. Share your favourite books, watch your favourite movies and play your favourite games.

When people want to be involved

If you are the dying person, *you get to share as little or as much as you wish with those you love.* You may feel that you need to protect your family from the harsh realities you are facing, but bear in mind that your family members may feel they want to be more involved. If you can, let them. When loved ones feel as though they are in the picture, they can more easily cope with what is a difficult situation for everyone.

John, 75, was suffering from an engorged spleen as an additional challenge to his terminal diagnosis, which prevented him from comfortably sitting or lying down. As his mobility decreased, his family found different ways to be with him that provided him with comfort and interest throughout the day.

His son would arrive at the same time each day to watch a particular TV program with him, and they both found comfort from this simple routine.

At the same time, John got very cross with people who wanted to ask about his illness – he had enough time to think about it during the long nights of insomnia. He wanted to think about other things in the daytime.

One of his happiest last moments was the afternoon when his young grandson sat with him and showed him his toy car collection, talking about every individual car and chatting about everything and anything. 'It really took me out of myself.'

How to make the tough decisions

Let's say you've got 'the diagnosis'.

Whatever it is, there will be choices you can make around how much treatment to have and how much it will improve the life you have left to live. Nobody is all that interested in becoming a statistic for medical science, if it means that they will spend their days hooked up to machines or in extreme discomfort.

Wall-staring as a hobby has never really taken off. BUT there are lots of great reasons that people choose to prolong their life beyond its natural course, from spending more time with family and grandchildren, to seeing your beloved team win a premiership.

The important thing is that *you choose.*

If it's your loved one who is in this situation, be guided by them. In talking through their condition, many people come to a realisation that the benefit they have been receiving from their medication has now been outweighed by the struggle of day-to-day living, and it's time to stop.

'Being allowed to die in a society which avoids talking about death, and where the dying process can be extended in unpleasant ways, can be harder than you think.'

Sarah Winch PhD

Fear clouds our judgement and can compromise our choices. Deciding to speak up, and discuss your death and your options, is not only the brave decision but will be extremely helpful.

What if I don't know what I want?

Most people haven't thought much about their own death. It can be confronting to think and talk about, especially when the choices are unclear. Remember you can sleep on any decision you feel uncomfortable about. Except in the most extreme circumstances, you will have time to make up your mind.

Start the process today and give yourself the best shot at getting clear on what you prefer.

Make sure those you love know how you feel about:

- *Where you would prefer to die, at home or in a care facility?*

- *Whether there are people you would like to see – or NOT see*

- *Whether there are rituals or rites you want performed*
- *What sounds, smells and sights you love*
- *Your companion animals, with you or not?*
- *Whether you mainly prefer TV and radio on or off*
- *What the most comfortable place and position is for you.*

Remember you can – and probably will – change your mind, so get used to telling people when you do.

Sometimes starting with a list of what you *don't* want will help you get clear on what you *do* want.

When the treatment is worse than the illness

At the pointy end of life, everything can become quite clear. There often comes a point where painful or distressing side effects make living life unbearable. If we can cut through the 'prolong life at all costs' attitude of some medical professionals, we have a shot at dying in peace, without too much distress.

We're so fortunate to be living in an age where people rarely 'die like flies' from contagious diseases. As a trade-off, we get to live longer, and our older bodies develop far more degenerative diseases.

We still die.

And while we can manage many (but not all) of these diseases, eventually you will die of something. It's a useful distinction to look at whether any treatment will improve your life situation, or simply just prolong it.

There are plenty of treatments out there that can delay the onset of illnesses, and when the disease progresses there are more and more drugs and treatments you can access. However, it's important to realise that many medications have destructive side effects, which may make the life you were living no longer possible.

'My Mum has always said she would never tell me if she had cancer, because she wouldn't want us to worry. But I'd hate to find out when she's in hospital that she had been suffering all this time.'

Ruby, 35

If you have a serious illness and are given the option of pursuing medical intervention, it can be easy to feel that you don't have a choice – but you do.

Ask yourself:

- *What/who am I living for?*
- *Can I comfortably do/see/be a part of what I love if I undertake this treatment?*
- *What will this treatment give me? More time? Less pain? Relief from pressure? Better digestion? Less side effects from something else?*

Beryl, 75, was a fit and active member of her community when she was diagnosed with a condition that meant that she had a 10% higher risk of stroke than usual. Efforts to treat her situation with medication landed her in hospital as her body rejected the drugs, and her liver became quite damaged. Rather than start a different course of treatment with new risks, she discussed with her doctor the possibility of trying to 'wait and see'. This turned out to be a good choice, as her liver was able to repair itself and her system stabilised. Her risk remained slightly elevated, and Beryl was aware that she was still at a higher risk of stroke, but she was able to resume her active life.

Things to ask your doctor/specialist/ medical practitioner:

- *How much longer could this treatment give me?*

- *Will this treatment cause other changes to my body?*

- *What side effects do I need to be prepared for?*

- *Will I need other medication to help my body survive this treatment?*

- *How will my current state of pain/discomfort/ disease change if I take this treatment?*

- *Can we discuss this again when I have had time to think this through?*

- *I need to … (see my team win, get to my birthday, finish my memoir) … can this treatment help me do that?*

- *How long can I safely put off making this decision?*

- *Is it vital that I start right away? What am I risking?*

- *How long will I be on this treatment for?*

The Brave Questions:

- *'Would you accept this treatment if you were in my shoes?'*

- *'What is the worst-case scenario if I choose to undergo the treatment?*

- *'What is the worst-case scenario if I choose not to have the treatment?*

What are the alternatives to this treatment?

Can I postpone treatment, and what effect would this have?

Would you accept this treatment if you were in my shoes?

Please bear in mind that you can always ask for a second opinion. Not everyone has the same approach in medicine. You aren't asking for anything that a competent medical practitioner wouldn't ask for themselves.

Time

You may have more of it than you think, but it's never a given. The number 37 bus could have my name on it this afternoon. (Spoiler – it didn't – but you get what I mean, right?)

While we all know that we won't live forever, and many of us don't accept the truth of it,

I'm here to tell you, we're all going to die.

Support at medical appointments

If you don't feel comfortable making these choices, or discussing them with your doctor, take along someone who can help you navigate the facts. This might be a close friend, family member or a death doula.

Remembering stuff like this is *hard*.

Whenever I have to have one of these conversations, I inevitably forget to ask something important. *Write things down in preparation. Take notes. Make recordings.*

How to support someone in a medical appointment

Dear support people,

You get to ask the questions that the person doing the dying can't but wants to. You're the one with the clear head. The backstop. They won't thank you for shielding them from the truth, even if it's uncomfortable.

I know that you are already having a tough time processing all of this, but you picked this book up, didn't you? That tells me you are prepared to do whatever it takes to help your person die as good a death as they can.

Maybe they will be fine and be able to navigate the discussion comfortably, or maybe they will be like most of us and freeze up with TMI (Too Much Information). Check out the questions above. You may need to be the one who does the asking.

If you can, have a cuppa with your dying person before the meeting with the team.

Find out what they need to know.

Find out how much risk they are comfortable with.

Find out which treatments they are happy to have, and which treatments are not on their OK list.

WRITE THIS STUFF DOWN AND TAKE IT WITH YOU TO THE APPOINTMENT.

Make as many notes as you can during the appointment or ask if you can record the meeting on your phone.

After the appointment, you may be able to write a short summary, which will help not only you and your dearly departing one, but friends and family if they are asking to be kept informed.

Making a group page on social media can help keep people informed. You can create a private Facebook Group, and only invite the friends and family members who need to be involved. Then you can post updates once, rather than sending out multiple messages. There are also websites which help you coordinate support with meals etc, if you're lucky enough to have a network around who want to help out.

Jean was an active 83-year-old woman who lived independently. She sang in her local choir and was well known and loved in her community. She had strong opinions on every aspect of her life (and the lives of others) and liked her living situation to be 'just so'. She was able to do her own cooking and shopping, could walk short distances by herself and was healthy for her age. A major stroke left her in hospital, unconscious and gradually deteriorating. The hospital offered the distressed extended family the option of surgery to relieve the pressure on her brain, which they accepted without hesitation.

The surgery gave Jean a return to consciousness with limited eyesight, slurred speech and no capacity to swallow, and the need for months of rehabilitation which she resented intensely. She spent twelve months in a wheelchair before another stroke rendered her unable to speak or eat at all. Her next eighteen months of life were in a small room in a high care facility, being fed via a stomach tube and with very little ability to communicate with her visitors or the staff caring for her.

While in the high care facility, Jean endured several bouts of pneumonia which her doctors successfully treated with antibiotics, each time leaving her in a more weakened state than before. Jean's relatives could see that this was not a life that she would have chosen for herself, and finally decided to ask the medical staff not to treat Jean's pneumonia and just keep her comfortable. A nephew sat by her bedside *and gently explained this to Jean, and after he left, she died peacefully that night.*

If you are the support person for someone with a terminal diagnosis, it is important that you listen to them. They may have never had an opinion beyond chocolate or vanilla in their life, but they will know what feels right to them at the time of dying and if they don't know, that is the time to ask for support from palliative support staff, death doulas and counsellors.

People also change their minds, and that is their right.

You, dear carer, don't have to make any of their decisions for them, especially if they have already discussed their advance care directive with you.

Keeping a Book

Should the person you care for become disorientated or non-verbal, a notebook by the bedside is a perfect way for friends and family to stay in touch and up to date. You (and any visitors) can make notes about who visited, what the medical state was at the time and what visitors did, whether it was play music, read poetry or the newspaper out loud, or just sit quietly with the dearly departing.

Keeping your own book

When you are caring for someone in those last, very intense days, whether it's at home or in hospital, keeping your own personal notes is so reassuring. Time stretches out and things become quite unreal. To be able to look back over your notes and recall why you made the choices you did can provide quite a lot of peace of mind in the final days.

You may not be thanked

If you're in this for accolades and glory, you might as well pack your bag right now. Being a support person for someone who is dying is about as mundane a thing as you can imagine, and the rewards are small – but potent.

Picture this: you're sitting at the bedside of your nearest and dearest, and they have finally breathed their last breath. Their death wasn't pretty, or particularly noteworthy, but it was dignified and as gentle as possible, and they felt cared for and supported. You got to give them a few small moments of comfort – revisiting good memories, a nice smell, some soothing sounds, some people they loved, and then they were gone.

For many people, that is reward enough.

But, dear support person, know that there will be moments of:

- *frustration with bureaucracies, machines, timing and people*

- *helplessness when you see your beloved one in pain, breathless or struggling*

- *anger when nothing seems to be going right*

- *grief because you know that at the end of this, there's no celebration.*

'*I said to him, "Dad, you're dying, mate." He didn't want to hear it. He told me (in his slurred speech) to piss off out of the room. It had been a long time since I had seen him that angry. If the stroke hadn't affected his arms, I'm pretty sure he would have up and punched me.*

I gave him a few moments, but when I went back in, I could see things had changed for him. That day, he told the doctors to stop all the treatments except the pain relief.

I was happy to be his support person, but I didn't sign up for the anger.'

Bruce, 44

Talking to children

Talking to children about someone dying

First of all, dear ones, there are a number of good resources out there that will give you more help in this difficult time, and I have listed some at the end of this book. Here are just a few tips to help you navigate a significant time in anyone's life.

If you're a parent and still shocked at the news of the impending death of someone you know, talking about it with your children is the one thing you wish you could put off. But trust me, it's never going to get easier. So while everything is raw and sad, be honest with your children. Make sure you use the words dead, died, death, rather than any of the multiple soft phrases that get trotted out when someone is dying. Once children feel like they are in the picture, they will be less anxious and less worried about what they have possibly imagined.

I don't promise that it will be easy. The tough stuff rarely is.

When someone is dying, children are likely to see adults in distress – not just the person dying, but those around them. Reassure them that this is what being sad looks like and that everyone is feeling sad in their own way.

Let them see some ways to comfort others who are in distress, whether it's with a hug, bringing tissues or a glass of water, or holding hands. It's best not to force a child to do any of these, but if they understand what's appropriate in the situation it will help them, especially if they see adults doing the same things.

In an ideal world, we live to a grand old age and die of complications from an ageing body. It's good to be able to explain to a child that 'grandpa died because his body was old.' It's understandable and gives children a perspective on death that's a bit more manageable for them – people get old, they die.

Someone who is younger and dying is a hard one for us to process, for all kinds of reasons. Make sure you are as clear as you can be and be prepared to be honest – you won't have all the answers, and nor should you expect to.

Talking to children about the death of their parent

Dear Dying Person,

When you speak to your children about your diagnosis, you don't need to go into *all* of the details.

What they need to know is what's likely to happen to you over the coming months, weeks, days.

They will need to know whether you are likely to be at home more or in care, on a respirator, not eating, gaining fluid, getting fat, getting thin, taking pain medication … the list goes on.

Someone else's illness is always a bit of a mystery, and more so for children who don't have the prior experience that many adults do. Of course, you'll need to tailor things to their age group – more mature children may want more facts. It might even be helpful to book a time in with a sympathetic doctor or hospice carer who can help you by filling in the blanks.

When your child knows what's happening, they can devote far more time and energy to spending time with you in a positive way.

If children don't know what's happening, they will find ways to ensure they are noticed, which probably won't be positive. Children act out when they feel unsettled.

Can they help?

If they know how they can help – according to their age – it can be a way for the family to feel more connected.

Children can:

- *Help cook and serve meals*
- *Pick flowers for the room*
- *Change the pictures on the walls for fresh ones*
- *Bring treats*
- *Tell stories*
- *Make tea/coffee*
- *Sing with you or for you*
- *Choose a good smell (eucalyptus, lemon, basil) to wipe down the room with*
- *Play your favourite song*

- *Give hand massages*
- *Bake*
- *Look through photo albums with you*
- *Read aloud – your favourite stories or theirs*
- *Manage the music playlist*
- *Play quietly on the floor*
- *Snuggle.*

Children have been known to think that they caused the illness that is killing their parent. It's so important that you reassure them that *it's not their fault.*

Remember what it is that you love doing with your children – and do that.

- *Friday night movies*
- *Baking*
- *Picnics*
- *Computer games*
- *Building things*
- *Board games*
- *Card games (the good old UNO)*
- *Gardening*
- *Watching sport on TV or IRL (In Real Life).*

If you don't have family traditions, you can always invent some. These are the times that your children will have to look back on once you're gone.

Children and the dying

When someone is in the last days of life, they may want to see children or grandchildren, or they may just want to remain very quiet and private. Find out what they want (if you can) and please respect those wishes.

If a child wants to visit but the dying person has asked for no visitors, the child can write or draw (or videotape) something for you to take instead.

If the dying person wants visitors but the child/children are not in the mood to be quiet or calm, it's unlikely to be a good match.

If you sense a child visitor getting agitated, distracted or bored, take them out of the room. Have a backup plan if you can, so the child can be otherwise entertained while you spend time with your loved one.

But sometimes, just sometimes, the stars align, and children can have a beautiful moment with a loved adult before they pass.

It's all individual.

The death of a baby

When a woman has been pregnant, but a baby does not survive for whatever reason, it is difficult for everyone involved. It's unbelievably sad.

Historically, when a baby who has died has been quietly removed with the minimum of fuss, the family can spend a lot of time grieving the loss of the child, always wondering where they were, and whether they did the right thing.

How to prepare yourself (as best you can):

- *Be gentle with yourself.*
- *If you know you will be giving birth to a child that has died, bring the clothes you plan to put them in. Plan to hold them, for as long as you need to, plan to bathe them and dress them.*

- *Think about how your extended family might need to be involved. Make a plan that includes them somehow.*

- *Plan to speak to your baby, sing to them, tell them about your family.*

- *You can have someone come and take pictures of you.*

- *Take hand or footprints if you wish.*

- *A naming or religious ceremony may feel appropriate to you.*

A death doula, and/or a caring funeral agency can be called in to support you through this time. There is no need for embalming or other complicated procedures. A funeral service can be held at the hospital, in a religious institution or at home if you prefer.

All kinds of pregnancies that end without a babe-in-arms cause grief. Find and get the support that you need, whether you are the parent, family member or grieving friend.

Remember that the best laid plans will change moment to moment according to what is possible.

Talking to terminally ill children

Dr Alan Wolfelt says, 'We show our love and respect for all children by being honest and open with them. We show our love and respect for dying children by helping them understand that they are dying.'

Children really do 'get it' when adults aren't honest with them. Like that 'Get Well Soon' card for someone with Stage 4 cancer, they see the huge inconsistencies and because they can't fathom why an adult would do what they are doing, they tend to get anxious and can act out.

A child who is dying – and who knows that they are dying – has the opportunity to deal with it in their own way. They may choose not to hear what has been told them – and that is their right. Often children will take the information in in little 'bites', sometimes asking for more information, and at other times sailing blithely past the stark reality of their situation.

As a parent, it is an almost impossible conversation for you to have with your child. But it is – potentially – the most important opportunity you will ever have to connect with your child.

Children have the capacity to hear and process what we tell them. If you're not sure you can be the one to tell them, have a team around you who can support you, and plan to have the conversation in the presence of a counsellor or medico who can fill in the gaps.

There will likely be questions that you can't answer. 'I don't know, but let's find out' is very reassuring for children, especially when you follow through with finding answers.

Anyone who has ever discussed anything with children will know they ask the most fascinating questions. It's OK not to know the answers, because you can always find out for them.

Remember to care for yourself as much as you can.

When you are dying, why are you staying?

- *Maybe you think you're not supposed to die.*
- *Maybe you didn't plan on dying until you got to a magic number: 90? 100?*
- *Maybe you think you're not allowed to die.*

Some people worry that their family won't be able to get along without them. And yes, when someone you love dies, it can feel impossibly hard.

Being upfront about what's going on – that someone is actually dying – can help make the situation a bit more bearable. Some people are better at this than others, whether friends and family or professionals. I've seen death doulas walk into a living room and talk death from the get-go, and the relief for all concerned is intense. People are often very relieved that someone has been able to approach what's going on with honesty and experience.

Making choices

Dad finally told the doctors to stop all the treatments. The moment he made that announcement, a weight seemed to come off him. It was like he had been carrying an expectation that he would get better, even though we all knew it wasn't possible. At 88, it was the right thing to do. The doctors, until that time, had been talking up rehab and therapy, but he couldn't even swallow, let alone really talk. His two favourite things in the world were yarning and eating, and they were promising a life where in all probability he couldn't do either. Nobody wanted him to suffer any longer but letting him go was tough.

Pete, 52

I've said it before and I will say it again – when you know you are dying, it's **your choice** how 'what comes next' is handled. If you're courageous enough to speak up and say what you need and want, particularly before talking and thinking becomes difficult, then those you love can help make that happen.

If you have discussed and developed an Advance Care Directive with those you love and your medical staff, then you will have made a positive contribution to what kind of conversations you can have when things get harder.

Making basic preparations: the bureaucracy surrounding death and dying

Dear dying person,

You are in a really good position *right now* to have a say in what happens to your things after you are gone. Maybe it's all the same to you, and you'll be quite OK with everything being boxed up and sent to charity. Or maybe there are some things you can make decisions about now which will mean that people you love:

1. Get to take care of things you care about, and

2. Don't have to make guesses about what you treasured (and didn't treasure) after you're gone.

3. Can help you in a practical way, whether helping you sort your things, tidying up your online profile,or making deliveries.

The Bottom Drawer Book by Lisa Herbert is a tremendous help in prompting you to make note of everything someone else will need after you have died.

Pets

Now is a good time to find someone to take care of your pets. They may not actually leave you until you die, but knowing that they will be taken care of can be such a comfort.

It's not a good idea to assume that they will just be taken care of – actually speak to the person you would like to take care of your animal(s) while you can and ask if it's possible. It is a huge commitment and some people just won't be able to do it, for whatever reason.

Try and avoid advertising on the internet if you can, but if you do, try and get someone you trust to inspect the 'good home' your pet is going to.

Pets are such a great source of comfort, so if at all possible, keep them with you as long as you can. A good foster carer will understand this and will help you keep your pet until they really can't be cared for any more by you or your carers. Hiring a dog walker, or a pet sitter to come in and manage the physical needs of your pet as you are dying, will mean that you will have the animal with you for much longer with fewer worries.

What is an Advance Care Directive and what can it do?

These days many states have laws surrounding Advance Care Directives. An Advance Care Directive is a document you complete in conjunction with your doctor while you are still able. You get to say which types of care you are happy to accept and which life-prolonging treatments you do not wish to have. This becomes important when you are in a position where you are no longer able to speak for yourself. Until then, you have a say in how you are cared for.

You will be asked to appoint a medical decision-maker who will be asked to make choices on your behalf should you be unable to. In Victoria, you can also appoint an official support person who can assist you to 'make, communicate and give effect to your medical treatment decisions'.

Make sure your medical decision maker knows where your ACD is stored.

The ACD can cover a wide variety of specifications, but ideally should provide guidance to a hospital or doctor on your wishes around medical procedures, such as whether you would wish to be resuscitated in the case of a heart attack, what you would prefer if you are unable to swallow, whether you would want intervention in the case of a severe stroke, and many other cases. Most GPs are happy to help a patient prepare their ACD, and it's often a good moment to find out your medical team's own opinions around treatments at end of life, and whether they are a good fit with your own.

You can add anything else to your ACD that you wish people to remember during your last days of care.

Like a birth plan, it's useful to have but can be difficult to follow when the realities of the situation become apparent. It's easier for people to do right by you when they have some understanding of what you value. And that, my friends, is what an Advance Care Directive can provide for you.

Make your will

Sounds simple, doesn't it? You know you are dying, so you make sure your will is in order. Which means we ALL should have a will. And look, even if you're not planning on dying, you should have a will. Just in case.

Dying without a will is called 'dying intestate' and even wealthy people such as Aretha Franklin do it. Why? Because nobody wants to accept that they could die. Around half of the Australian population doesn't yet have a will. Preparing a will, choosing an executor who can carry out your wishes and letting them know that you have chosen them, is key to a smooth 'sorting out'. Make sure your executor knows where your will is stored, and make sure they will have access to all of your accounts and passwords.

Give your executor a copy of your current information and remember to keep it up to date.

Making a will doesn't have to be complex. There are only a few formalities a will needs to have, to make it legitimate. You can obtain legal will kits from newsagents, but should get legal advice if:

- *You have a beneficiary who has special needs*
- *You have property or assets overseas*
- *You want to specifically leave someone out of your will*
- *You have a trust or private company*
- *You have patents, special licences or have written books that will earn income after you die*
- *You are ill, in hospital or are older*
- *You have children to different partners.*

Make a will. Please.

Your digital profile

Do you do your banking online?

What about Spotify? Netflix? Subscriptions to special software?

What do you want to happen to your Facebook account after you die? You can nominate a digital representative to manage your social media accounts when you have died, and they can either close your account down or set it up as a memorial to you – whichever you prefer. But you need to let them know what you want.

Passwords

What are your important passwords, and how often do you change them? How do you remember them? Do you have them written down and stored somewhere safe?

Even if you don't store most of your passwords, please *ensure your executor has your email password on hand*. This could be written into the will and stored in the lawyer's safe storage. This is vital because just about all other programs can retrieve a lost password via your email address.

Your 'stuff'

You may not feel like it, you may not be physically up to it, but the more 'stuff' you can let go of before you die, the easier it will be for your family after you go. Those car parts, books, excess televisions and clothes are all surplus to your needs now, and you certainly won't need them once you have died. So, if you can, find a home for them. Or get a rubbish removalist in. Many of them will find homes for your goods rather than send it all straight to the dump. Ask when you book.

Many people find great comfort in gifting their treasures before they die. If you have some special treasures, make sure you have written down who they are to go to. Or hand them to your loved ones while you can.

If you are caring for someone who is dying, let them lead. Our stuff is important to us. Having a say in what happens to it is possibly one of the only things your loved one has any control over at the moment. Just make sure you know where their will is, and how to access their digital profile.

Another word to the grieving – don't feel you have to give everything to charity straight away. The bereaved can get a great deal of comfort from a few personal items, and there are beautiful creative ways to treat beloved items of clothing to create precious mementoes.

What happens afterwards

Do you want to have a say in how your funeral is conducted? Do you want a traditional funeral according to the beliefs of your family and culture? Do you want something different? Now is the time to have a think, and a chat, about what you would want to happen.

Almost everyone has heard a eulogy where 'they've got it wrong'. **Write your own eulogy** if you want them to get the facts straight. Get someone you trust to write it down and make sure the funeral arrangers know where it is.

Even if you have no particular requests or funeral plans, your loved ones will appreciate knowing this. It makes their choices much less of a burden.

The way funerals are being conducted is changing, and you may like to investigate:

- *Green funerals and burials*
- *Burials, composting, cremation and other possibilities*
- *Living wakes*
- *Keeping vigil after death*
- *Whether to embalm or not*
- *Shrouds, coffins and caskets, including cardboard coffins.*

Support services for the dying

What *is* palliative care?

Palliative care is a brilliant service, and once you find out that you are 'on the fast track', get on to them. People can access palliative care for a very long time, as it's all about supporting quality of life, for however long that may be. Your palliative care service will help you manage medications and side effects and help ensure that you get the best quality of life, for however long that might be.

Some people will have better access to palliative care than others, simply because of where they live. Many rural areas have only a small 'pal care' team, so you'll need to do a bit of homework to find out what is available in your area.

Your palliative care team will be able to help you decide what support you need and give you an idea of what is possible.

Until you or someone you love is dying, chances are you won't know what's even on offer.

What is hospice care?

Hospice care is available for people whose illness is expected to cause death within six months. Some health practitioners use the terms 'palliative care' and 'hospice care' interchangeably, but palliative care tends to be longer-ranging and includes life-extending treatments. Hospice care tends to focus on comfort and alleviation of symptoms as far as possible, as well as supporting you in the way you approach death and dying.

There are a few dedicated (usually private) hospice facilities in this country, but much of the hospice care as practiced in Australia is based in people's homes, using dedicated hospice staff.

Voluntary Assisted Dying

In some parts of some countries, euthanasia, or Voluntary Assisted Dying (VAD) has been made legal. The safeguards around the legislation are very strict. Check with your doctor (or organisations such as Go Gentle Australia) to establish whether Voluntary Assisted Dying is accessible where you live. Voluntary Assisted Dying has very strict guidelines surrounding its application, so if you think you might wish to access it, make your enquiries early, while you are able.

I was able to support my uncle as he requested and got access to Voluntary Assisted Dying. Life had become so hard for him – every day was painful, even with an increase in meds. Even breathing was a struggle. The doctor felt he wasn't going to die any time soon, so his immediate future was hellish. He often said, 'Why can't they just take me down the back paddock and shoot me?' He had been a farmer all his life and had had to end the suffering of many animals over the years.

I sat by him as he took the medicine, and he drifted off peacefully. It was a gentle death, a kindness really, and I was very humbled to be able to do this for him. I was so relieved that his suffering had ended. I wouldn't have done it any other way.

Joyce, 59

Dying at home

The circumstances surrounding dying are often likened to childbirth. It's messy, there are plenty of variables and every single one is different. At the same time, there are some cues and stages that everyone has heard of, even if they don't really understand them.

Unlike childbirth, the end isn't usually a bundle of joy.

Unlike childbirth, it can go on for a very. long. time.

More people these days choose to die at home, with plenty of support from medical teams. It is very disruptive to normal home life but can be immensely comforting to the dying and their carers.

As a carer, it is vital that you arrange support and care for yourself, whether it's quiet time away from the sickroom, a regular coffee with a counsellor or empathetic friend, or physical support such as getting a massage or doing enough exercise. Your entire body and mind will be under constant pressure and you will need to timetable your days to ensure you get adequate self-care time. Speak to your support team to work out how to make this happen.

Deathbed care

Whether you are choosing to die at home, or in a hospital, there are some elements of deathbed care that it's good to be aware of. If you know what is possible, then you will be able to say what you prefer and what you definitely do not want.

There are lots of professional manuals out there on deathbed care, and ideally you will be cared for by a team which includes trained personnel. Pain relief and wound care are things you will need to discuss with your medical team.

What you'll find here are some ideas for your friends and family, to help you know what will help and what will hinder. Keeping the lines of communication open between friends and professionals will make things easier for everyone.

Once a person is 'on their deathbed', the focus needs to be on keeping them comfortable. Life-prolonging treatments can be kept to a minimum (or possibly stopped altogether unless the dying person has a specific wish). Treatments to ease suffering and pain need to be brought to the fore.

Washing

You may be feeling very uncomfortable about having someone else wash you. Rest assured, it's a perfectly normal thing to do, and humans have been doing it for centuries. For many carers, it's an honour to be able to support the one they love this way. Besides, a wash and freshen up is one of the nicest things you can have done for you when you are stuck in bed. If you have a favourite soap or smell, please let your carers know, whether you're at home or in care. It can feel so restful to be freshly washed and smelling 'right'.

Linen change

If you've ever seen a bed being made while the person is still in it, you'll realise what a handy skill it is. There are YouTube videos that show you how. Fresh linen makes a huge difference to a person's wellbeing, as long as the changing doesn't distress them too much. Problems with skin as well as internal organ pressure need to be considered before a bed change is attempted.

In-bed comfort

Once you're at the stage of being in bed all of the time, you'll realise how great an alternating-pressure air topper can be on your mattress, particularly if your skin isn't very stable. Don't feel that you shouldn't ask for one, as bed sores can make life miserable – and avoiding misery and making life as good as it can be is our goal here.

Other people swear by sheep skins, memory foam and gel mattress toppers. If you have the chance to try them out before things get difficult, you'll know which one feels most comfortable.

Smells, fragrances and the like

This is a highly individual thing, and some people are far more sensitive to smell than others. How does the room smell? Could it do with some fresh air?

If fresh air isn't possible (because it's too cold or windy outside, or you're in an interior room) what else can you do to make the smell pleasant?

Be careful of flowers – some, like lilies, can have an overwhelming scent that will leave everyone more agitated. Roses are generally a good bet – change the water daily to ensure it doesn't go smelly.

Often this is **not** the time to use supermarket air fresheners as they can cause headaches, and because the dying person is usually confined to their room, they end up breathing in far more of the air freshener than any of the visitors, which their failing organs can find it very difficult to process and get rid of.

Equally, essential oils can be too overwhelming at this time, so if you plan to use them, consult a qualified aromatherapist. Less is usually more at this stage.

Some novel air freshening ideas:

- *Crush fresh herbs in the room: mint, rosemary, or lavender are good.*

- *Crush eucalyptus leaves, pine needles or lemon scented gum leaves.*

- *Break open freshly baked bread.*

- *If your patient likes a particular type of herbal tea, brew some and leave it to steam on the bedside table.*

- *Cooking vanilla (not air freshener vanilla) in warm water can be spritzed or wiped around the bed.*

- *Some light spritzers like Australian Bush Flower Essences 'Space Clearing' or 'Transition' essences can provide a lot of freshening without adding intense perfume.*

Light and sight

As a person is dying, lights tend to be dimmed as they can become highly sensitive to light. It's important to know what you prefer while you are able to say so, to help you stay comfortable.

Do you sleep best in a darkened room? Do you need some light? Do you like curtains open or closed?

Taste

A basic part of the care of someone who is dying is keeping their mouth and lips moist. There are hospital swabs for this process, but for many, swabbing with familiar liquids such as cooled tea, soft drinks or juices is far more comforting than the pharmaceutical swab product and helps them connect to pleasant memories. Watch out for mouth ulcers when swabbing.

Lip balms are also very useful as your lips will dry out, and it is lovely if you can use a lip balm that you are familiar with.

Noise

Unnecessary noise can be very disturbing to a dying person. Soothing sounds, on the other hand, can have a relaxing effect on everyone in the room.

Noises you *may* be able to minimise include:

- *Medical machinery*
- *Movement around the building*
- *Televisions and radios*
- *Mobile phone 'pings' and 'beeps'*
- *Ringing phones (they can be taken off the hook, turned down or even unplugged in the case of hospital phones)*
- *Visitor noise (limit the number to minimise noise)*
- *Rattling fans*
- *Ticking clocks*
- *Unnecessary conversation.*

Carers, don't be afraid to ask to move outside a hospital room for long explanations once the dying person is not participating in the discussion. The sense of hearing operates whether we are conscious or not, and a bit of awareness around the sounds the dying person is exposed to can make life more comfortable for everyone.

There are plenty of sounds which can help distract you from discomfort and pain. Soothing sounds which you can specify to have by your deathbed:

- *A quietly playing radio or television*

- *A playlist of your favourite music*
- *Live music if you have musical family members*
- *Someone singing for you*
- *Friends reminiscing*
- *Rain or ocean sounds (YouTube has several eight-hour recordings of these sounds)*
- *Guided meditations.*

The Threshold Choir is a movement which began in the US in 1990 and is now available in many communities in Australia. They are a group of volunteers who sing a curated repertoire of music designed specifically to soothe pain and calm the dying. They can be invited to sing at the bedside of private individuals and visit many hospices and hospitals.

Some hospitals also have music therapists. It's worth asking about, as music played and sung live really does have positive benefits, from pain relief to lowering blood pressure and relieving anxiety.

**You may never have had someone sing
to – and for – you before.**

Now is a very good time to change that.

Pets

Many people have a beloved pet who will be wondering what has happened to their human. Pet visits to hospital and hospice can be possible, especially for well-behaved dogs. Talk to your health care team about arranging a visit. Many hospitals have special animals who visit.

When someone is dying at home, pets will be able to come in and out, with supervision. They can be a great comfort.

Deathbed cues

Experienced medical staff can often tell when a person is moving into the final stages of dying.

These stages don't progress in a 'check-the-box' fashion, but it is helpful to know what the cues might be, and what to look out for.

Body temperature, vagueness/lucidity, having visions and changes to facial features are all very normal stages. There are great resources available which will give you more details on the final stages. And your professional support people will be only too happy to answer your questions in this regard.

Self-care when you are the carer

Whether someone you love is dying at home or in care, it's so difficult. You will struggle with all kinds of emotions, as well as the day-to-day practicalities of supporting someone who is dying. Added to that, the situation can change from moment to moment, so you need to be able to function as if you were in a high-powered managerial job that ran 24 hours a day for an unknown length of time.

You will need to care for yourself, as much as for the dying person, so that you can stay the course. It's a marathon of uncertain length. You need good sleep, good nutrition, your own health support, someone to give you a break, things to bring you joy and a way to debrief. Every day.

Changes in family dynamics

Often, when a family member is dying, there will be some member of the family who just isn't coping. They may deny what's happening, insist that the dying person gets a different treatment, pick fights, or generally just make life difficult for the carers around the dying person.

Keeping stress and angst to a minimum in what is already a high stress environment is a must.

1. *Subscribe to the theory that you only ever bail the water OUT of the sinking ship. Let them dump elsewhere. Get them some support, if they will let you. Keep that room as peaceful and harmonious as you can.*

2. *Hand them this book.*

3. *Sometimes, this person may be you. If you work this out, find a way to decompress. Get out of the house/hospital/hospice and go find something that helps you let off steam.*

Good choices for carers:

- *Going for a walk*
- *Drinking fresh water*
- *Sitting in a café and reading*
- *Writing a journal*

- *Meditating, yoga, tai chi*
- *Visiting someone you trust and asking them to hear you out*
- *Hanging out with children doing fun stuff together*
- *Sitting in a cinema (popcorn optional)*
- *Getting a massage/reiki/acupuncture/physical treatment*
- *Letting someone else do the early morning/late night shifts and getting some sleep.*

Poor choices for carers:

- *Picking fights*
- *Trying to get the dying person to apologise for past behaviour*
- *Staying up late*
- *Making assumptions about your dying person's wishes*
- *Making assumptions about the medical state of your dying person*
- *Eating all the sweet treats at once*
- *Drinking to excess*
- *Any situation where you don't get to move your body for more than 24 hours.*

Are you currently struggling as a carer?

Do something that will bring joy to someone else. Studies have shown that an easy way to increase your own happiness is to bring happiness to someone else. Buy someone a coffee, make a donation to a charity you think could do with a hand, or pay for someone's groceries. It's surprising how much of a mood lifter it really is.

> **'I'm actually rather romantic – and here is my idea of romance; you will soon be dead. Life will sometimes seem long and tough, and god, it's tiring. And you will sometimes be happy and sometimes sad, and then you'll be old, and then you'll be dead.'**
>
> Tim Minchin

So there you have it. Dying. We all do it.

I hope this book is the start of a conversation that will make your end-of-life a more open, loving, courageous and supported process.

Die well, my friends.

Testament

When you hear that I am dying

Don't rush about

Sit a minute and feel me in your core

Know that I will still be there before, during and after

When you hear that I am dying

Know that I am on a sacred schedule

Just as you are, and always have been

When you see that I am dying

Don't hold my hand too long

Sing to me

Play me beautiful sounds

Tell me the old stories

Let me hold my cat

Lie beside me and lean in

And let me be, too.

When I am dead, don't clean my fingernails

Wipe my face – that's nice –

Wash my quiet heart with your tears

But leave my fingernails to show the next life where
my joy was

in the mess of creating

the muck of the Earth

Show me that the time for these trivial gestures of civilisation is over

When I am dead

Find a quiet place you can gather

Whoever wants to come

Please sing

Please dance, a little

Smile that I was

And give what's left to the Earth

So I can help feed the souls to come.

Amanda Collins

Useful resources

On children and death

- For pre-school children https://iview.abc.net.au/show/play-school-beginnings-and-endings/video/CK1913H001S00

- An excellent article by Dr Alan Wolfelt is available at www.griefwords.com, entitled Helping a Child Who Is Dying.

- Glenn Ringtved (2001) Cry, Heart, But Never Break, Mem Fox (1999), Sophie

For teens

- Molly Carlile (2010) *Sometimes Life Sucks: When someone you love dies*

On supporting those you love as they are dying

- Margaret Rice (2019), *A Good Death* (Australian)

- Katy Butler (2019), *The Art of Dying Well* (US)

- https://takethemameal.com/

Personal stories of death and dying

- www.memoleaves.com

- Michelle Bourke (2017), *Conversations with Paul*

Keeping a personal record – being prepared

- Lisa Herbert (2013), *The Bottom Drawer Book*

- Lyndsay Lowe (2014), *Life and Beyond, Instructions for my family*

Other useful references

- www.advancecareplanning.org.au

- https://deathcafe.com/

- http://palliativecare.org.au/

- https://www.betterhealth.vic.gov.au/health/ServicesAndSupport/voluntary-assisted-dying

- https://www.australia.gov.au/information-and-services/family-and-community/wills-and-powers-of-attorney/wills

- https://www.gogentleaustralia.org.au/

On clearing your home before you die

- www.sorted.net.au

- Margareta Magnusson, (2017), *The Gentle Art of Death Cleaning*

- Karen Kingston, (2017), *Clear your Clutter with Feng Shui*

"Testament" by Amanda Collins originally published in N-Scribe 14, November 2019

Acknowledgements

Debra Luccio

Helen Bramley Jackson

Annie Tsernjavski

Lissanne Oliver

Kitty Wiggett

Heather Munro

Rose Munro

Deb Wain

Dave Munro

Blaise van Hecke

Busybird Publishing

About the author

Amanda Collins is a poet-singer-songwriter with an interest in all aspects of human life. After a childhood on the river plains of the Goulburn, she now divides her time between two hills – one on Taungurung country and another one on Wurundjeri land. She can often be found talking about death and dying, poetry and creativity, and making soundscapes with a variety of instruments including crystal singing bowls.